PERSPECTIVES IN MOTION AND STILLNESS

PERSPECTIVES IN MOTION AND STILLNESS

Inspired Commentary on T'ai Chi and Meditation

by Steve Ridley

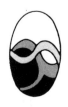

Good Karma Publishing, Inc.
Fort Yates 1996

Copyright © 1989 Steve Ridley
All rights reserved. No part of this book may be reproduced, stored in or introduced into a retrieval system, or transmitted in any form or by any means (electronic, mechanical, photocopying, recording or otherwise) without prior written permission of the publisher.

GOOD KARMA PUBLISHING, INC., Publisher
P.O. Box 511
Fort Yates, ND 58538

Printed in the United States of America by BookMasters, Inc., Mansfield, OH

First Edition, 1989
Second Edition, Revised 1991
Third Edition, Revised 1996

Cover design, drawings and nature photographs by Steve Ridley

Contributing photographers: Harper Bookman, Lia Ridley, Renee Wilson

Design and layout by Jean Katus

♻ *Text printed on recycled paper*

Library of Congress Catalog Card Number 95-82363

ISBN 1-882290-01-1

Dedicated to my parents
KEN AND HOPE RIDLEY
in appreciation of their selfless love
and enthusiastic support
through the years.

CONTENTS

Foreword xi

Introduction 3

T'ai Chi Perspectives 5

T'ai Chi Poetry 33

Meditative Perspectives 51

Meditative Poetry 71
   Observations of Nature 73
   Internal Observations 81

Author's Note 89

Appendix 91
   General Meditation Instruction 93
   Tan T'ien Meditation 95
   Meditation to Awaken the Heart Center 97

FOREWORD

Aptly titled, *Perspectives in Motion and Stillness* presents a personal commentary on T'ai Chi and meditation, blending the balance of what moves with what is still in the varied experience of these inner arts. Though the authentically-inspired writing comes from Steve Ridley's regular involvement with these disciplines, anyone who practices either or both of them will immediately recognize a universality in the way he has expressed himself through the statements and poetry. By the same token, anyone who has not experienced T'ai Chi or meditation can also identify with the beauty and truth that manifest through the simply and directly voiced words that come straight from the heart.

Sometimes very practical and reminiscent of the daily challenges we all face, other times esoteric and operating at a level that requires deep study of our inner selves and how we experience Reality, the writings offer a wide range of ideas to contemplate and reflect upon many times over. And that is what makes this book so exciting! It contains pieces for everyone to benefit from, whether one is a beginner on the spiritual journey or whether one has been led that way for a long time. From the serious to the playful, from observations of life in nature to inner insights, from the personal to the universal, Steve has succeeded in illustrating what the potential of each one of us truly *is*—if we can but allow our inner awareness full expression in the material world.

Steve Ridley is certainly well-qualified to share his thoughts in *Perspectives in Motion and Stillness*. He has been studying T'ai Chi and Yoga since 1975. He practices T'ai Chi Chih and T'ai Chi Ch'uan daily, along with Kriya Yoga Meditation. His two main teachers are T'ai Chi Master Justin F. Stone and Yoga Master Roy Eugene Davis. The former appointed him as the Spiritual Head of T'ai Chi Chih, and Mr. Davis trained and ordained him to be a representative of the Kriya Yoga lineage.

Steve conducts workshops and retreats in T'ai Chi and meditation throughout the U.S. and Canada and leads several T'ai Chi Chih teacher accreditation courses each year. He provides on-going instruction in T'ai Chi and meditation in Denver, Colorado where he also works as a jazz drummer and massage practitioner. In addition, he offers group meditation sessions weekly in his home and gives presentations for holistic health organizations and New Thought churches.

Steve is not new to writing. He frequently writes articles on T'ai Chi and meditation and has produced two inspirational books and a T'ai Chi Chih videotape. Nearly all of what appears in this book has not been previously published.

I feel sure that you who read and savor the pieces in this volume will find your life—inner and outer—much enriched, as mine has been. Steve has been a teacher to me, as well as a loyal friend. Through the profound statements and poetry in this book, you, too, can experience his gentle teaching and advice.

Jean Katus
Fort Yates, ND

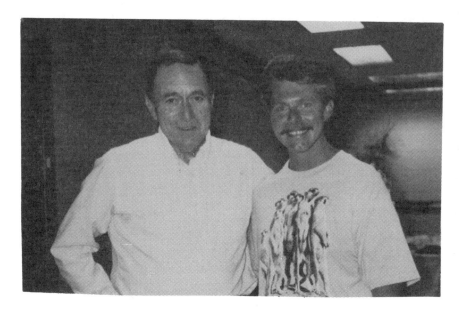

Justin Stone (left), developer of T'ai Chi Chih, with the author

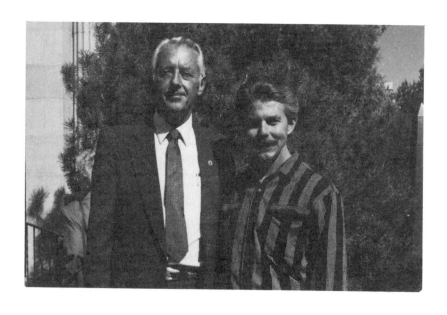

Roy Eugene Davis (left), Kriya Yoga Master, the author's meditation Preceptor

INTRODUCTION

T'ai Chi and Meditation have enriched my life, and through this book I am sharing some insights and inspirations that occurred through the practice of these subtle disciplines. I hope you will find confirmations of your own experiences, support for your continued involvement with T'ai Chi and/ or Meditation, and useful direction for progressive refinement and benefit in these arts.

I have found that T'ai Chi and Meditation complement each other. Following T'ai Chi practice, it can be beneficial to be still, in order to direct full attention inward, toward absorption in the silent center of our Being. Conversely, after deep interior absorption, the practice of T'ai Chi movements can provide grounding and the synchronization of mind and body, which helps integrate the transcendental perspective of Meditation.

The statements and free-form poetry presented here are best digested in a contemplative manner, perhaps after a session of T'ai Chi or Meditation practice. Each writing was naturally derived from individual periods of practice with these arts. The poems and statements are not contrived, nor are they rehashings of others' perceptions. It is impossible to directly convey authentic and transpersonal realizations through words, yet I have tried to capture something of the original insights through each statement and poem.

There are many useful systems of T'ai Chi practice and many effective approaches to Meditation. We are naturally attracted to the methods that serve us best. Regardless of the specific techniques and formats, the underlying purpose for engaging in these arts is identical: the actualization of WHOLENESS.

May this humble offering assist your quest for Enlightenment and Self-Actualization in some way.

                                            Steve Ridley
                                            June 12, 1989
                                            Denver, Colorado

T'AI CHI PERSPECTIVES

Though several systems of T'ai Chi practice exist, the ultimate aim of each is to establish the practitioner in harmonious living, while developing the innate potentials of the mind-body. There is no superior T'ai Chi form. A wise master once explained that the technique and the art are the least things to be concerned with. He was alluding to the Essence of T'ai Chi practice, which is not contained by form, format, belief or doctrine, but which can be known and lived from. In this context, T'ai Chi practice systems can be likened to an assortment of equivalent inlets to the Ultimate Resolution. Pride in one's chosen practice formula indicates immaturity and limited perception.

Who can master T'ai Chi, the Power that orders the universe? The best we can do is accord with T'ai Chi, the "Supreme Ultimate," through trust. When we feel separate from a thing, there can be no "mastery." When our identity *is* T'ai Chi, all striving ceases. The individual seed unfolds its potential and becomes the tree, which is diversified and unified in its expression of T'ai Chi. Mastery is *knowing* the infinite within the finite.

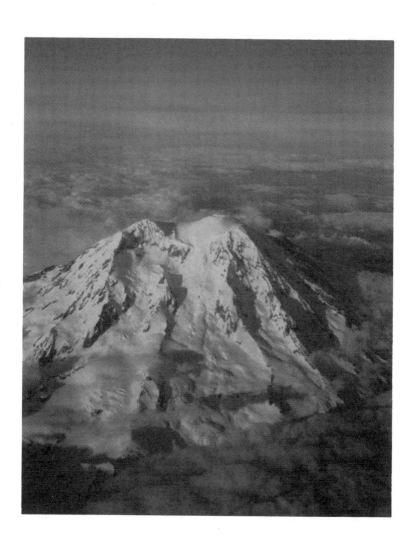

T'ai Chi practice refines our physical awareness in progressively subtle ways. Not only do our balance, agility and posture improve, but our capacity for sensitive perception throughout the collective physical system also increases. A novice would be astounded by the deeply intimate and comprehensive physical awareness and attentiveness of a mature T'ai Chi practitioner. Through the regular study and performance of T'ai Chi, we become acutely conscious of subtle changes in structural alignment; muscular emphasis; tactile sensitivity; weight displacement; the cooperative relationships of the feet, waist and hands; and the correct anticipation that guides and transforms the postures through their related phases, in consort with a constant center. The beauty of this art is that it can never be fully perfected and that it fosters a process of continual discovery.

O

The most beneficial consequence of practicing any T'ai Chi system, regardless of how complex or simple, is that it makes possible the ordering of the mind-body in such a way that Original Consciousness can manifest.

O

Daily involvement with T'ai Chi practice re-orders our internal constitution and enlarges our capacity for perceptiveness and contentment. Physically we become resilient and supple, fortified by the effective circulation and accumulation of chi. Mentally we become highly sensitive to internal and external processes and are capable of regulating them in the interest of balance and harmony. Spiritually we are continually awake in the unconditioned freedom of Being, while enacting specific and creative functions within the context of yin-yang interactions. T'ai Chi practice develops Ultimate Integration.

O

T'ai Chi practice reveals that there is a universal energy that mobilizes all processes, and that it is possible to improve our alignment with its life-affirming impulse. To the degree we are successful in our alignment, we know fulfillment.

To perfect alignment and apply the desired emphasis for the optimum functioning of each posture and transitional movement, we can assume stillness at various points in order to adjust the weight displacement, degree of relaxation and the positioning of the torso and limbs. By stopping to adjust the alignment and emphasis in this way, eventually all movements will be enacted effortlessly with power, grace and stability. An extreme application of this would be to occasionally utilize a primary posture for standing meditation practice. By enduring in a particular stance for several minutes, overall strength is fostered, chi fortifies the body, subtle aspects of the position are understood and meditative clarity can unfold.

O

In T'ai Chi practice the body must be unified through synchronization of motion. Without proper synchronization and coordination, the chi flow is interrupted, jarred, weakened, and loses its momentum. Of main importance is the unification of chi flow through the feet, legs and waist. This is primary and provides the effective foundation whereby chi may be specifically directed and shaped through the various circular patterns expressed by the hands.

O

An important aspect of T'ai Chi practice is the component of circularity. This principle of movement contributes to the efficient distribution, development and accumulation of chi in the body. Throughout the enactment of postures, we create circles, ovals and ellipses, connected by supportive curves and spirals so that chi is continually activated, increased and contained. If we overextend, straighten or stiffen, we contribute to the stagnation, weakening or dissipation of chi. The hands should be slightly cupped, the shoulders slightly rounded, the chest slightly concaved, the abdomen slightly convexed and the joints unlocked. A rounded area tends to attract and control chi, while a straight area tends to have the opposite capacity and influence. The curved shapes of all life forms and the cyclic patterns of nature's processes demonstrate the life-generating principle of circularity.

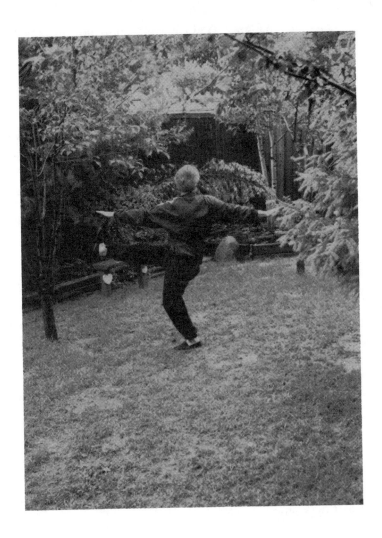

The tan t'ien is the balance point in the body, through which all T'ai Chi movements originate and return. It is the psychic plexus where chi is generated and collected, and from which chi is directed. Many T'ai Chi practitioners keep a continual focus of feeling within this abdominal center, which cultivates and matures the chi, increasing its volume and potency. Deep internalized meditation on the tan t'ien can be beneficial.

As we practice the art of T'ai Chi, perfecting movements through ideal alignment, fluidity, and continuity of internal attitude, chi expresses more efficiently and completely through us and we become vital conduits for the manifestation of harmony in our world.

O

T'ai Chi is a Spiritually-based discipline and ultimately a way of life. We are first attracted to the practice by its flowing, graceful postures and the magnetic physical power it generates. As our understanding and practice mature, we begin to recognize the Spiritual foundation of the art.

O

While performing T'ai Chi movements, we expend the least amount of psychic and physiological effort, so that chi is easily circulated, controlled and absorbed. We open the soles of the feet to drink in the chi of Earth, soften the gaze and relax internal dialogue to receive the chi of Heaven, allowing the power of integration to fully manifest.

O

T'ai Chi cannot be mastered. The best we can do is to refine our enactment of the art and live according to our clarity of perception.

O

Persistence and patience are the foundation of T'ai Chi practice, much like the character of a river as it shapes and polishes its stones. In T'ai Chi living, the moment is sufficient and complete and patience is enacted naturally.

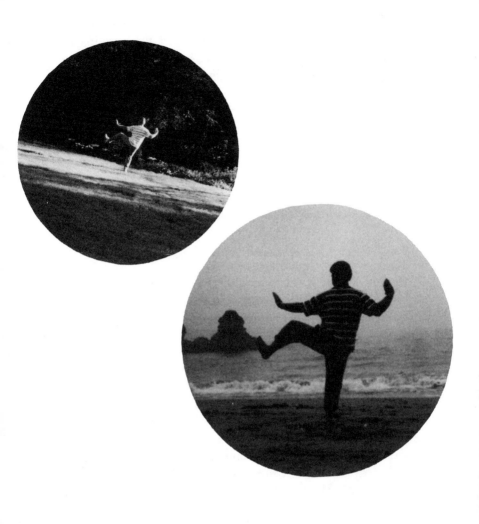

The beauty of T'ai Chi philosophy and practice is that application is continuous, whether performing forms or relating spontaneously. The value of T'ai Chi living is in the continual restoration of harmony it provides. The approach to mastery of T'ai Chi is demonstrated by one's capacity for living harmoniously within and without.

By realizing the true art of T'ai Chi living, we better accord with the spontaneous yin-yang cycles that arise. T'ai Chi living requires full awareness meeting each situation. Any useful action performed with utmost attention is, in effect, the practice of T'ai Chi. Formal practice of forms awakens us to the formless T'ai Chi. Discovering the formless T'ai Chi, all involvements are conducted effortlessly.

O

Through T'ai Chi involvement, we learn to internally harmonize yin-chi and yang-chi, which enables us to facilitate and manifest harmony as required by the on-going process of living. That Essence, which makes the play of opposites possible, continually inspires harmony.

O

The complementary and antagonistic interactions of yin-chi and yang-chi continually form and re-form as the underlying mobile energy blueprints that maintain creation. The separation and blending of yin-chi and yang-chi accomplish the complex and interconnected variations of motion and rest that are symbolized by the physical universe. Similarly, in T'ai Chi practice, the performance of movement variations requires that we distinguish yin-chi from yang-chi and that we also unite them. We differentiate yin-chi from yang-chi through interrelated, multifaceted combinations of empty and full, soft and hard, sinking and lifting, circling in and circling out, withdrawing and extending, closing and opening, etc. We achieve degrees of stillness, and ultimately realize undifferentiated Being.

Extreme yin-chi transforms into yang-chi, and when yang-chi reaches its utmost expression, it naturally converts into yin-chi. This process manifests continually in the cyclic flows of nature and is symbolically enacted and applied in a practical way through T'ai Chi forms.

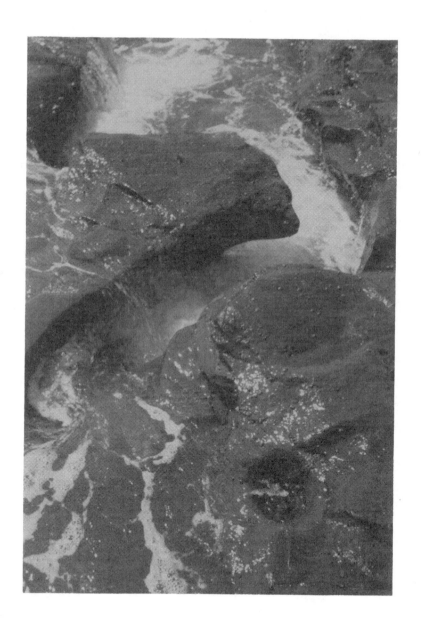

T'ai Chi practice activates self-transformation, according to the degree of intensity we apply. Exceptional students of T'ai Chi make rapid progress through consolidated application.

O

Through regular and correct practice of T'ai Chi, we are literally made over. We undergo a refining process that manifests as progressive Wellness.

O

As we approach our formal practice of T'ai Chi, it can be much like greeting a wise friend and mentor, from whom we receive needed insights and uplift. This "friend" imparts harmony and leads our awareness into the realization of integrity, stability and joy. We become more sensitive to the flow of Life-Force within and around us, as pursuit of mental fluctuations gives way to conscious clarity. Through our practice, we assist the on-going process of self-evolution by activating and balancing chi, the evolutionary energy. Self-evolution can be seen as the unfolding of our innate Perfection, and the development of chi quickens this predestined process. By cultivating chi, we accelerate the actualization of innate Perfection, which accomplishes the dissolution of suffering and reveals conditionless contentment.

O

The realization that we are essentially products of chi instantly renders us humble and grateful. From this recognition, our Universal Identity can be known.

In T'ai Chi practice, consistency and patient endurance are essential ingredients for success. By performing T'ai Chi movements, internal energy flows are re-ordered. Specific changes in the vibratory oscillations of internal energy, chi, occur in response to the execution of various postures and transitional movements. This beneficial re-ordering of the internal chi circulation has a direct, transforming influence on the functioning of the mind-body. Through regular practice, we effect a consistent patterning of internal energy flows, which develop in potency through time. By promoting the on-going generation of specific, life-enhancing patterns of chi circulation, we literally remake ourselves.

O

Though we endeavor to perform the T'ai Chi movements in an exacting and perfect manner, our perception and sensitivity are not contracted. T'ai Chi involvement fosters greater perception and sensitivity, an enlargement or expansion of awareness and capabilities for accomplishment. While performing the particular movement patterns or interacting spontaneously as we live the principles of T'ai Chi, we are focused on detail as well as the overall picture, simultaneously. We develop the innate capacity for living wholly, including all, while appropriately expressing our individuality.

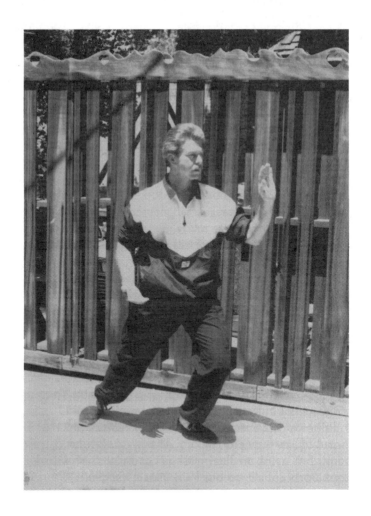

Through correct practice of T'ai Chi, one can attain exceptional health while realizing inner Certainty because the increased volume of circulating chi brings heightened vitality to the entire physiology, and the harmonization of it restores mental clarity and emotional stability. Chi directly influences the mind-body, and over time, through T'ai Chi practice, causes refinement, modification and personal transformation (evolution).

When we recognize that all physical systems are perpetually nourished and sustained by the circulation of chi, it becomes evident that physiological health directly reflects the quality of this circulation. Through T'ai Chi practice, we apply specific thought-movement patterns to encourage the optimum flow of chi.

O

T'ai Chi practice leads us from the temporary states of satisfaction and dissatisfaction to the Stable. Integrity is developed, which provides enduring Stability greater expression through the mind-body.

O

In T'ai Chi practice it is essential to maintain an equal receptivity of the Great Yang force from above and the Great Yin force from below, by emphasizing the sensation of "rootedness" in the soles of the feet and the sensation of openness in the crown of the head. In this way the Great Yang force and the Great Yin force are combined and incorporated harmoniously.

The action of sinking and lifting alternate and combine throughout the sequence of movements. In order to rise properly, we must be rooted below, and we are able to sink effectively when we are lightly suspended from above. This north-south polarity is kept in balance to create a harmonious wedding of the two forces. By cultivating this important principle, we are likely to experience harmony and fulfillment, living in poise and stability amidst changing circumstances because we are able to rise and fall with equality and ease as necessary.

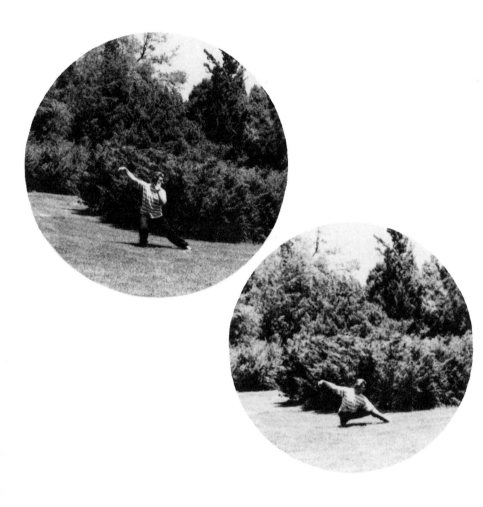

Practice of T'ai Chi becomes consistent and ultimately represents our essential vocation, regardless of the type of work we render.

T'ai Chi is a way of life that continually cultivates harmony through equanimity and ever-centeredness. Each thought and action become spontaneous T'ai Chi practice when we are ideally oriented. The true foundation of T'ai Chi involvement is our ever-evolving relationship (partnership) with the Essence of life. Being established in authentic understanding of the Essence governing all processes, we are able to harmonize and accord with diversity, without being distracted by the commonly-pursued modes of pleasure-pain, gain-loss living.

O

The beauty of T'ai Chi practice is that it fosters the revelation of the Essence upon which it is based. Practicing correctly, as advised by a competent teacher, we become knowers of this Essence.

O

Serenity in the midst of changes is an attribute that is cultivated through T'ai Chi practice. When we are established in changeless Peace, regardless of what transpires, a major objective has been achieved. In this state of serenity, designated "good" and "bad" blend in equanimity.

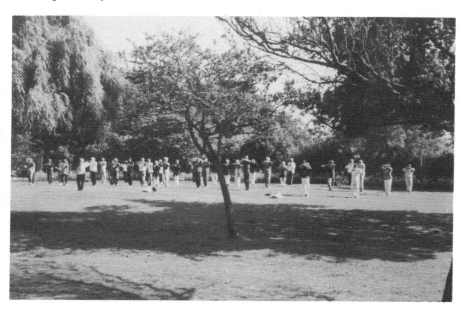

T'ai Chi practice becomes Meditation when we realize ideal synchronization of focused thought and action. In this state we perceive beyond the relative mixing of postures in motion and know the contentment of non-striving Wholeness or conditionless Joy.

O

In T'ai Chi practice we release and gain, gain and release, while established in conditionless Equanimity. T'ai Chi practice leads us back to this Equanimity, which is not diminished by the appearance of gain and release.

O

Through involvement with T'ai Chi forms, we recognize the nature of yin-yang interactions: cause becomes effect, which initiates cause, and so on. It is a perpetual cyclic action, seen as endless streams of motion, continually re-forming as cause and effect.

O

Perceiving nature and its subtle cyclic patterns, relationships and processes, we begin to discern the underlying functioning of chi, the wisdom-guided force, as it prompts and enlivens all manifestations toward completion and fulfillment of purpose. Recognizing chi as the inexhaustible agent that continually nourishes and regulates all life processes in all universes (fine to gross), we begin to comprehend its Source.

O

Yin and Yang mutually provide assistance for each others' expression through the fundamental nature of their characters—one cannot exist without the other. The interdependent relationship is symbolized and creatively manifested in T'ai Chi practice, and it is the primary foundation upon which the art was formulated. The operation of this complementary polarization is the relative essence that empowers T'ai Chi forms and guides self-unification. The persistent contemplation of the characteristics of yin and yang at play in nature and continually forming as the universe results in progressive enlightenment.

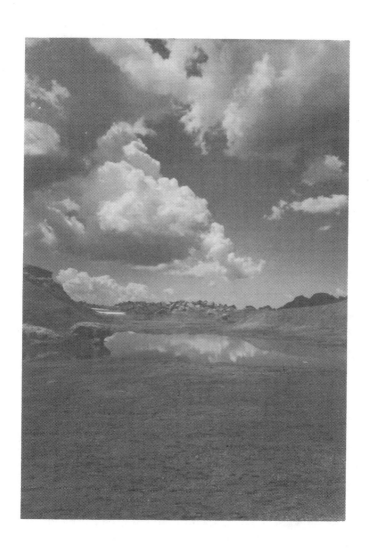

T'ai Chi practice might be referred to as a physical approach to Spirituality. By performing the art with sensitive physical attunement or full awareness of movement continuity and power of alignment, mental equanimity results, allowing Original Clarity to function more completely.

O

The character of the "Great T'ai Chi" is demonstrated through the application of softness and continuity. Continuity is that which is unceasing and devoid of fragmentation. Softness is that which is yielding and therefore enduring. By living in softness and continuity, Universal Energy expresses through us in dynamic and useful ways.

O

In T'ai Chi practice we move with relaxed integration, being continually open or vulnerable, and thereby absorbent, pliable and enduringly stable. We blend with and embrace all things, finding equanimity and limitless strength. It is basically a matter of self-surrender and a willingness to enlarge our capacity. Through faithful practice we develop.

O

T'ai Chi warriors cultivate inner stability amidst the changing scenes and perceptions that continually occur. T'ai Chi practice is a profound method for coming to terms with the changing. When we practice regularly and well, we manifest the "T'ai Chi Nature," which provides continuous fortification in the face of instability.

O

T'ai Chi practice is a process of learning to abide in the center while employing the opposite characters of yin and yang in a fluid manner, by blending and distinguishing these two forces. Through mental direction, the chi flow is guided and the symbology of postures is enacted to accomplish the desired balancing. This practice cultivates the capacity to interact spontaneously and usefully in natural circumstances as they arise. Abiding in the center, we are capable of embodying and expressing aggression (yang), reception (yin), and differing combinations of these modes, without being seduced by or overly invested in any mode of character we are required to enact for the sake of balance.

Through T'ai Chi practice, we invite universal energy, or chi, to express in greater volume through us. We learn to regulate and cooperate with this evolutionary force. By performing the T'ai Chi movements properly, we learn to accord with the life-affirming impulse of chi, thereby fostering self-transformation, improved functioning, creativity, vitality, wisdom and joy.

O

A constant principle of T'ai Chi is the dynamic cyclical activity of expansion and contraction and the transition from one to the other, as seen in the cycle of seasons: winter = extreme yin; spring = yin joining yang; summer = extreme yang; fall = yang joining yin. All T'ai Chi movements demonstrate this basic cycle of gathering and extending, which assists the generation and circulation of chi. By understanding the cyclic nature common to everything and everyone, we can discern the stable, unifying Essence supporting and directing all cycles.

O

In movement, softness and continuity are embodied as faithfully as possible. It is essential that we move in a unified manner with power and steadiness, through every pattern and subtle change, creating an underlying emphasis of equality and balance. If we embody the flowing character of a great river and are as responsive and agile as a cloud being mobilized and sculpted by wind, we will assist in the more complete nourishment of the mind-body by allowing chi to accomplish every action. As we continue to develop this refined synchronicity of motion and internal openness, we manifest enduring strength effortlessly. By working patiently and continually with T'ai Chi, including the study and application of its profound life-enhancing principles, T'ai Chi is able to work for us, quickening the process of self-evolution, which ultimately culminates in liberation of consciousness.

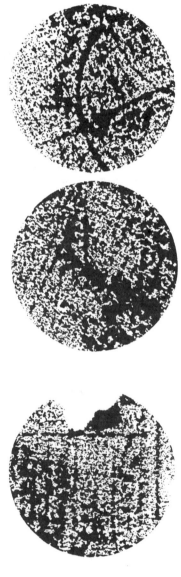

Cycles of Yin and Yang

Ink Print by Steve Ridley

T'ai Chi practice is a process that helps reveal the Unity and Peace that endures, beyond the reduced perception of chronic identification with mental conditionings. We begin to see through the mask of mortality and are gradually restored to our innate, conscious relationship with the "Grand T'ai Chi."

O

T'ai Chi or "Supreme Ultimate" sustains and encompasses the ongoing manifestation and activity of yin-chi and yang-chi, appearing as the totality of life's countless appearances and processes. The closer we are able to accord with T'ai Chi, the more we know harmony and fulfillment, regardless of the particular appearances and situations that arise.

O

Through the practice of T'ai Chi, we come to know ourselves more completely. By striving to perfect the movements, we cultivate the awareness of ourselves as Essence or Being. T'ai Chi forms are not perfected until Essence is the sole director, and when this is accomplished, formal practice becomes unnecessary, though it may be performed according to required direction.

O

Eventually, sincere practitioners of T'ai Chi discover something of the Essence of the practice, which is vastly superior to the particular forms and movement sequences. Ultimately, we pass beyond the fluctuating mental fetters that continually bind perception, and we are able to comprehend, more completely, the endless worlds of yin and yang.

O

By performing T'ai Chi forms correctly, we provide a favorable internal environment for the optimum expression of chi. The circulation and blending of this evolutionary force, through T'ai Chi practice on a consistent basis, quickens the process of personal development by activating and maturing all innate potentials.

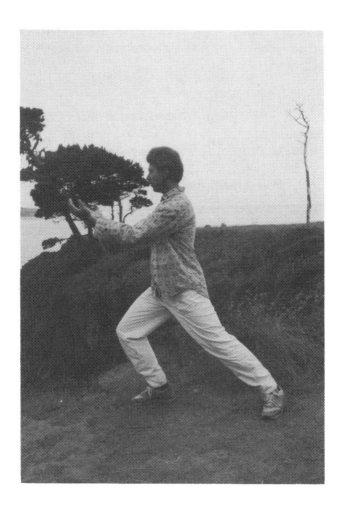

    In T'ai Chi practice we learn to abide in the enduring, changeless Center of dynamic strength and contentment, while creatively responding to the spontaneous, cyclic flow of life. Within the unpredictable cycles and sub-cycles of yin and yang, we are able to contribute useful directions and supportive influences, while being stably rooted in formless T'ai Chi. Rooted in formless T'ai Chi, we recognize that all that arises is supported by an inexhaustible stream of love.

T'ai Chi Master Justin Stone advises that there are two things to accomplish: "Know who and what you are. Accord with impermanence. You cannot accomplish the second until you have accomplished the first." When these two things are accomplished, we are liberated. This accomplishment is the true aim of T'ai Chi practice. It can be called the "Great Circle of Completion." Knowing our Actual Identity is half of the circle. Living in the world while established in our Actual Identity is the completion of the circle. In this state of awareness we know our Authentic Nature, beyond the operations of yin and yang (the play of opposites), and we are able to live harmoniously within the framework of yin and yang or "impermanence" because our outlook is comprehensive.

O

When we are able to lose ourselves in T'ai Chi practice, devoting full attention, Meditation is naturally born. The form gives way to the formless.

O

There are a variety of static poses in addition to the moving T'ai Chi forms. Prior to movement we are still, without thought, providing a neutral foundation from which to enter practice. Following movement practice, we can maintain a standing posture, to allow the generated chi to fully fortify the body and contribute to its reserves.

Mental performance of T'ai Chi forms can be a valuable involvement for sharpening and strengthening our power of concentration. It can also contribute to the refinement of postures and transitional moves, and directly influences the harmonization of chi throughout the body. Mental practice can consist of the systematic repetition of single movements or segments of the form in order to highlight subtle details of alignment and other spatial distinctions or more generally, the performance of the complete series of movements can be created. The most beneficial results are realized by entering into the process with full absorption, by applying visualization and sensory assimilation (feeling), making the exercise as tangible and realistic as possible. Mental T'ai Chi practice can be utilized while sitting quietly with eyes closed or prior to sleep.

Some T'ai Chi teachers are accomplished movement technicians and are perhaps even well-versed in philosophy, yet have little internal comprehension of the art. Nonetheless, they are able to convey the movement patterns accurately, enabling students to continue to practice on their own, to whatever degree of personal dedication, with the possibility of intuitively discovering the underlying, subtle principles upon which the art is based. The most complete type of teacher is capable of transmitting the Essence of T'ai Chi, in addition to giving detailed instruction in the performance of movement formats. Dedicated students diligently prepare themselves in order to attract such a teacher and to be able to openly receive the spiritual transmission that is offered.

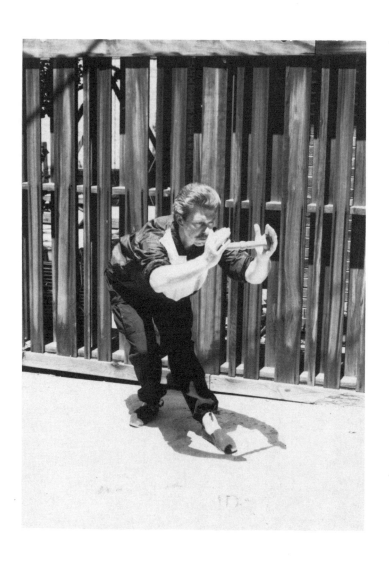

T'AI CHI POETRY

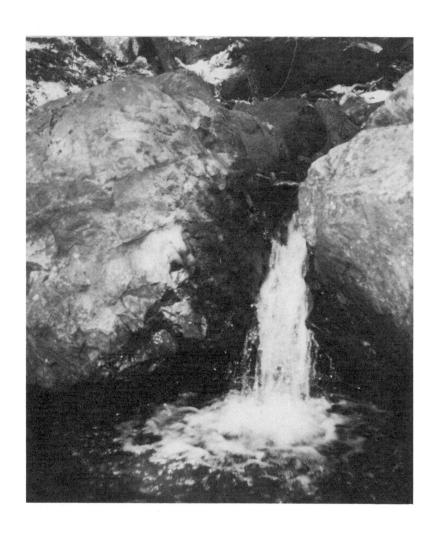

Early morning T'ai Chi practice
Beneath the old spruce,
Feeling reverence

Fresh delicate rain mist,
Sparrows singing spring

Within
The Cosmic Consciousness Pose
Love rings through every cell

Remembering Master Stone.

———

    Surrendering in practice
    Without rushing,
    Cultivating patience

      Listening in newness . . .
      Insights flash!

      Thousands of beginnings
      Dissolve growing pains
      Into Completeness.

———

Secure snowy blankets hush earth . . .
In the stillness of winter chill
Unconscious chimes vibrate air,
Warming T'ai Chi forms

Luminous rays shyly funnel onto Earth
Lifting vaporous scintillating swirls
Above warrior pines cloaked in white

Meditating, the whole world meditates . . .
Gratitude swells the heart and the world is joy-filled

An Awakening! Enlightenment flashes through all minds . . .
The collective BEING bathed in Sacredness!

———

Drawing circles in air,
Foolishness?

Moving in gentle unity,
Joy breathes

Earthen symphonies
Issue and transform

Why cling?

—·—·—

        Emerging—establishing—returning
        Each strives

        Amidst rising and rooting
        Without distinguishing

        One life gives
        Perpetual birth and death

        Impermanence is
        The beauty
        Of passing clouds

        Forever is
        The joy
        Of that witnessing ONE.

        —·—·—

Lulled into harmony . . .
New mind, astride motion

Chi-intelligence,
Condensing—radiating

Light at the top
Attunement.

———

    The division of interests
    Between heaven and earth
    Is humanity

    Worshiping yang and yin,
    Discontent conceals joy

    In the face of the One Life
    Re-cognition breathes joy!

    ———

Slowness . . .
Internalized . . .

Methodical rhythmic softening
Coaxes vibrant joy

Integrated motion reveals
STILLNESS!

———

    Connecting movements . . .
    One form

    Striving into stillness . . .
    No form

    Softness and continuity
    Reveal contentment

    Dynamic serenity
    Sustains and embraces all.

    ———

Above desire-driven pathways,
Behind boisterous mind-storms

T'ai Chi directs hearts
Infallibly toward freedom

A manifesting wholeness
Fostered in dispassion

T'ai Chi revives . . .
All will see anew.

Mountaintop serenity
Amidst the clamor . . .
Self-assertion-suffering

The eternal search,
The sacred promise

A joy-flower sprouts,
Nourished in T'ai Chi soil.

—·—·—

                        Body motions stir
                        Transforming meditations

                        Penetrating power
                        Enlivens the marrow

                        A linking with joy . . .
                        River of abundance!

—·—·—

Crashing waves re-form . . .
Effortless fluid motion

Aggression—release,
Life within life
Blending yin and yang

Slow unfolding harmony . . .
Seconds into aeons

In self-forgetting
T'ai Chi is known.

—·—·—

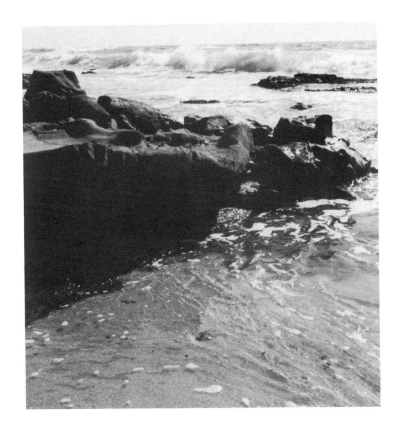

Fluid motion ease,
Soft orbiting hands dissolve

Withdrawn in movement,
Joy continuity . . .

Renewal,
No fight.

The most distant star . . .
Chi connection

Collecting opposites,
Roaming shoreless energy seas
Pleading liberation

Wave-ocean unity
Reflects the Eternal Center

Standing firm
In T'ai Chi freedom . . .
Soles of the feet!

———

        Within T'ai Chi
          · slowing, into self-nurturing

        Ease-full rhythmic blending . . .
          power unification

        Aligned through heaven and earth,
          greeting all directions

        The Heart of motion
          resolves every impression . . .
          peace perspective.

———

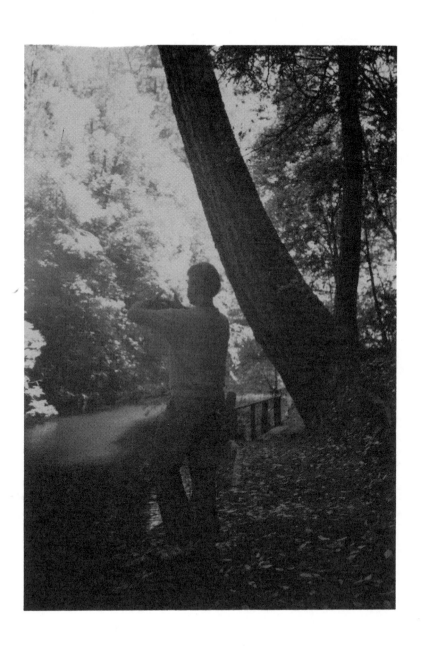

Formless T'ai Chi
Indwells form

Ancients taught:
Form is least important

Knowledge of form
Leads to internal stability

Consistent practice
Awakens chi, integrates diversity
And resolves into ONE

More and more effortlessly,
Our world inherits joy.

—·—·—

                Through countless faces
                T'ai Chi knows wholeness

                Bestowing, transforming,
                Integrating, awakening . . .

                Within the Great T'ai Chi
                Lights and shadows dance.

                —·—·—

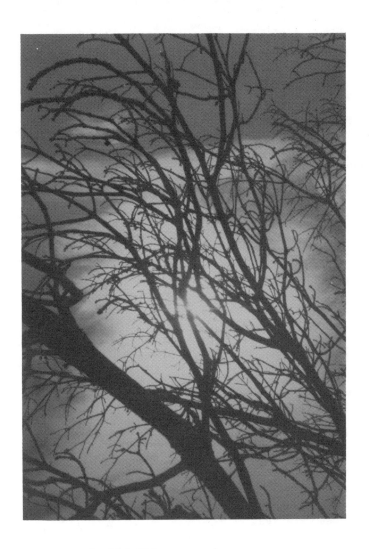

In T'ai Chi communion . . .
The universal pulse thrives,
Lighting every heart

Known—unknown,
We create—we withdraw

Recognizing . . .
Vanity dissolves.

Awareness flowing
Through worlds of thought

T'ai Chi peace and vitality
Erase restlessness,
Soothing and emancipating

Clarity . . .
Being within doing.

―.―.―

                  Front to back
                  Side to side . . .
                  Who moves?

                  Each action,
                  A prayer of gratitude

                  Through cycles
                  to INFINITY!

                  ―.―.―

Insubstantial—substantial,
Pivot and revolve,
Fading in—fading out

Thoughts turn
Toward the ONE

Deepening Center . . .
Formless resolution.

―.―.―

                  Slooow T'ai Chi
                  Into early grey mist

                  Trees, lawn and stones blend, shiny wet
                  Reflecting a Westerner, cloud-like
                  Breathing comfort and grace
                  Softly from the Heart.

                  ―.―.―

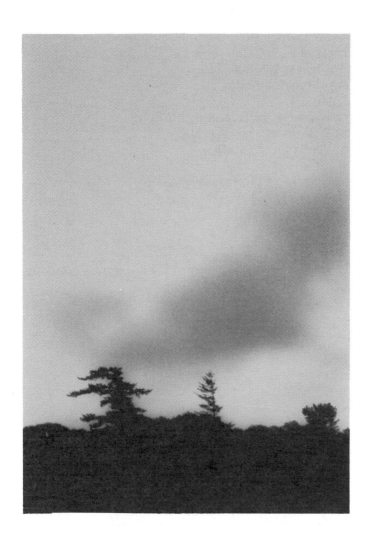

In the open quiet
Of stillness in motion
Birds sing, wind blows, clouds sail . . .
Unification impresses the Heart.

The Great T'ai Chi

I am the ever loving ONE,
The nurturer of each living form
And the boundless intelligence
Expressing through all minds

The universe has its birth and death in ME,
I am ever with those who seek ME
And with those who shun ME

Residing evermore in the cave of your Heart
I alone am your dearest friend
And certain guide . . .

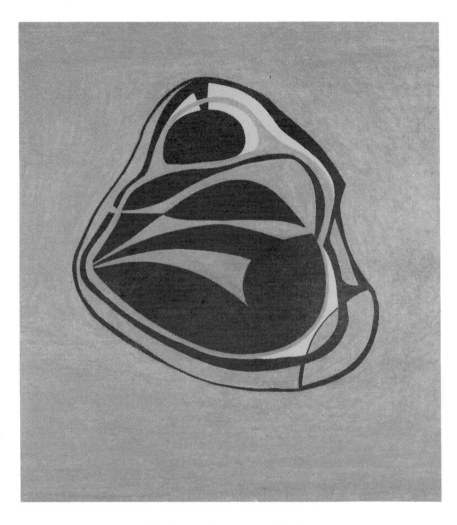

Meditator Resting in Wholeness
Pencil Drawing by Steve Ridley

MEDITATIVE PERSPECTIVES

Meditation practice is a very subtle internal art that leads progressively to the undifferentiated state of Wholeness or Being. Though various methods of mental focus and breath regulation are employed, all valid meditation approaches eventually resolve into the direct realization of Being. This illumined state is innate to every person, and through the practice of meditation, this Original Consciousness is remembered.

O

A spiritual person is one who lives in accord with Reality, existing moment by moment in the recognition of Reality. Spirituality is not a specific conceptual outlook, supported by belief structures or faith in doctrinal formats. When there is actual recognition of Reality, conceptual information about Reality is naturally abandoned.

O

Forms and formulas of meditation practice assist us in providing the condition through which Original Consciousness is revealed (remembered). Meditation practice is similar to the actions of the wind and vaporization process that clear the morning fog, revealing the perpetual sun.

O

We are multidimensional beings, existing simultaneously within many levels of expression, ranging from fine to gross. We are the Original Consciousness animating and existing through these interdependent realms of expression, though we are essentially changeless and formless.

O

In meditation practice internal focus is essential. The convergence of one's whole attention, of one's entire being, within a single space, will lead to the absorption that reveals Meditation.

53

Authentic spiritual literature carries the power of knowing, which was realized by the author. The words were carefully chosen to most faithfully convey the original revelations that flashed through the mind. By deeply contemplating the subtle written sharing of enlightened beings, direct spiritual insights can unfold. This is very different from the process of ascribing to another's assertions by believing what has been presented. Through the thorough contemplation of enlightened commentary, our own innate knowing is resurrected.

O

The inspired writings of illumined beings can, in turn, inspire us to awaken to our innate clarity of Being. If we have yet to rediscover our Full Identity—above (in addition to) thought processes, sensory input and emotional states—we can begin to sincerely contemplate the subtle meaning and thrust behind the shared words of enlightened authors, past and present. They impart their liberated awareness through selected language to assist us in recalling our ultimate Fulfillment.

O

From the meditative perspective, the basis of true learning stems from quiescence. All knowledge unfolds from within us. By listening carefully, we allow all expressions of life to be our preceptors. In relative, conditioned awareness, we recognize things by our classification of them. By quieting our mental activity, we are able to see things as they are and to experience original learning. In meditative clarity we recognize the Authenticity of everything.

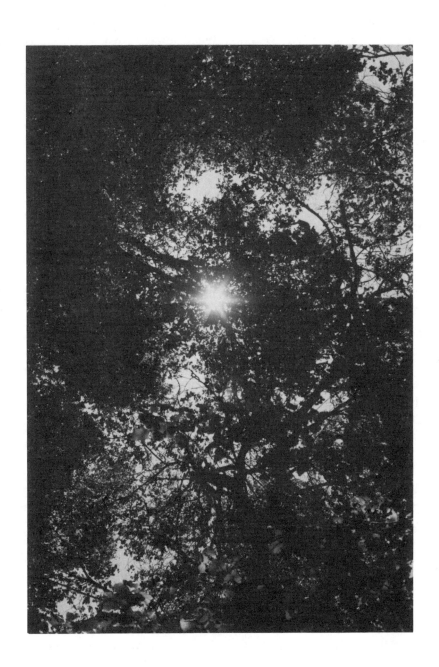

Sitting still with closed eyes may appear to be self-contraction and world-withdrawal to the uninitiated, yet the Meditative State is one of exceedingly sensitive perception, clarity and extensive awareness. When mental activity predominates with continually churning thoughts, our sensitivity becomes dulled and our capacity for perception is very limited. In this condition our awareness is boxed in, and the possibility of peace and fulfillment seem remote. The practice of meditation provides relief from this often chronic state of mental agitation, and, in time, Meditative Awareness can dominate, even while the most exacting work is being performed. At this stage, the Meditative State, cultivated through isolated practice, becomes a perpetual way of living.

O

The enlightenment path is a process of awakening to the clarity of Whole Awareness, rather than striving to conform to conceptual ideals of "spirituality."

O

The realization of our Imperishable Identity is a potentially liberating insight. In such clarity, the mind and body are recognized as extraordinary mediums through which we experience and interact in order to communicate and share the life-affirming substance of our Being. After this revelation, mind and body no longer dominate our self-definition, but are known as transitory agents that we sustain and live through, to assist the evolutionary thrust of life's creative processes.

O

Deep daily meditation can profoundly assist our efforts to break free of the mental boundaries we have constructed. The concepts we harbor tend to contribute to our acceptance of limitation. By clinging to conceptual constructs, we stifle potential creativity, the possibility of gaining unique insights and the ultimate manifestation of innate Wholeness. If we truly yearn for liberation, the release of all conceptual supports (belief systems and imagined securities) is imperative.

O

All experiences are potentially limitless adventures in Consciousness, filtered through our present capacity of perception.

Meditation is the ointment that heals a thousand woes. The mind-body continuum is soothed, saturated and bathed in Radiant Power which energizes, cleanses and opens one's subtle perception. There is no greater or more worthwhile involvement than the practice of meditation.

O

All hunger is essentially spiritual hunger, and all suffering is due to spiritual forgetfulness. At the root of all seeking is Knowing, and within continual hunger is complete Nourishment.

O

The initial challenge for meditators is to neutralize the predominant mental characteristic of desiring stimulation through diversity. Once this tendency is relaxed and replaced by one-pointed flowing of attention toward the object of meditation (visual symbol, mantra, or energy plexus), the only remaining obstacle, other than fleeting subconscious impressions that may arise, is our deep-seated reluctance to let go in self-surrender, which is closely related to our fear of death. Only by abandoning the immediate mind-body orientation can our Original Consciousness be known. As it turns out, the realization of Original Consciousness is one of expansive awareness, rather than the anticipated self-annihilation!

O

In meditation practice we undergo a progressive process of physical relaxation, mental quiescence and self-surrender (opening to the Larger Life). The "meditation experience" can be a source of true revelation that results in self-transformation. Resistance and unknowing during the initial stages of practice are transmuted into refined perceptiveness and the dawning of innate Wisdom. We recognize that illumination and perpetual fulfillment effortlessly spring from Being.

O

By attempting to fulfill desires, born through feelings of lack, satisfaction will always be incomplete. In the certain clarity of stillness, we recall our innate, enduring Fulfillment that is without cause.

The quality of Consciousness that we live from is shared with all those with whom we relate. It is what we contribute to our world and it is reflected in the way we interact. More important than the type of work we render is the state of consciousness that we impart.

The peace realized through meditative stillness is dynamic and all-inclusive. It instantly banishes feelings of anxiety, confusion and suffering; and introduces calmness, certainty and contentment. Peace is ever available and can be received and incorporated at any time. Meditation practice is the inlet for peace.

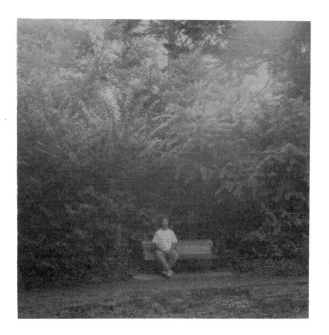

True Integrity is the foundation of wellness, fulfillment and power. Until we are established in spiritual Integrity or living in Wholeness, every thought and action will carry a measure of self-interest and the desire for fulfillment because we feel incomplete in some way. It is said that a Sage's most formidable strength springs from Integrity, meaning that the united harmony of spirit, mind and body allow unrestricted creative expression, intuitive functioning and dynamic physical endurance.

Wholeness ("holiness") is embraced by stilling the body and persistently emptying oneself into a stream of one-pointed surrender. Through steady dedication in this manner, regardless of distractions that may arise, one can realize the ultimate success of being Complete. This is the goal of all enlightenment ways.

O

By transcending the relative perspective of good versus bad, likes and dislikes, we can see through the limitless eye of Wholeness, which is all-inclusive and consumes any former impulse to find fault or favor, unduly manipulate circumstances or to pray for preconceived results. Through this illumined clarity, the most profound prayer is naturally offered because all visions of limitation have vanished.

O

Most pray with the hope of freeing themselves from various forms of challenge and distress. This common use of prayer is usually regarded as a last resort attempt to transform conditions. We tend to pray when we are overwhelmed by circumstances and emotional surges of discomfort. Prayer can be used to remove restrictions from the mind, to clear the way for Meditative Clarity, which brings renewal and strength and reveals the deeper meaning of conditions and circumstances. The ultimate prayer might be: "Let my ignorance vanish and my innate, Comprehensive Sight be restored."

O

Meditative clarity reveals the inner certainty of being essentially Limitless and ever Complete. In this knowing conditional limitations vanish. We recognize how they arise and why they are created, yet we understand that they have no lasting validity. Similarly, we recognize that passing clouds do not diminish the sun's brightness.

Meditation practice is meant to enlarge our capacity for conscious awareness or increase our clarity of perception. Ideally, the practice brings an expansive, comprehensive appreciation of self and life.

Beholding the changeless Essence within the transitory is true discernment and wisdom. In the alert stillness of Meditation this recognition is natural.

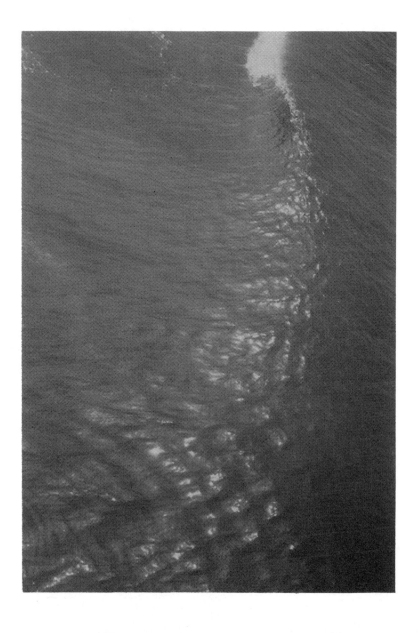

So-called virtuous conduct is natural and effortless when we live from the center of Reality. In this state of Clarity one *cannot* deviate from virtue. When our orientation is centered in relativity, we may attempt to cultivate and practice righteous behavior as a concept to be achieved. When Reality-based, we *are* virtue in action.

O

Everything is changing and ever new. There is an intelligent, benevolent stream of Creative Power behind this activity. The transitory individualized forms of this life, continually manifesting and undergoing transformation, are crystallized thought patterns that symbolically represent the Creative Power that shapes, sustains and evolves them.

O

Consciousness is ever pure and complete, yet when individualized and operating through and as the mind-body continuum, restrictions of various types arise. This is a transitory, surface condition that has no lasting reality or independence. Consciousness is never in need of liberation, though within the temporary condition of individualized awareness, the impulse of desiring freedom is experienced. Consciousness identifies so fully with the relative, individualized viewpoint it has assumed that the illusion of limitation occurs. A portion of Consciousness has forsaken Its naturally unlimited capacity in order to perpetuate the myth of separateness and limitation. When an individualized portion of Consciousness is restored to its natural state, through the individual perspective It created, we say that the person has *attained* Enlightenment!

O

The mind and body are inseparable and can be discerned as a unified continuum composed of creative energy. The mind-body is the contact or focal point through which Original Consciousness operates while relating to the material universe.

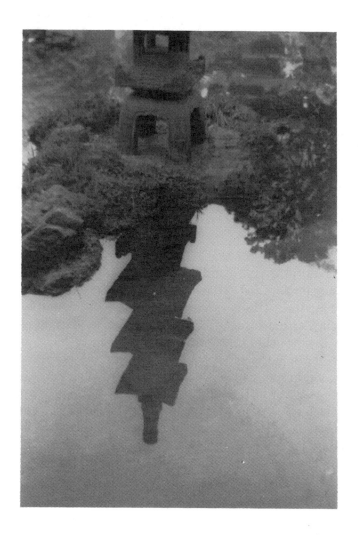

When we accord with Reality, we *are* Reality in expression. When we experience discord, we are not representing the potential thrust of Reality, yet Reality is ever expressing as us!

That which is subject to modification is a temporary, transitory extension of the one all-inclusive Reality, and is not independent and self-perpetuating. The agency that prompts various manifestations and orders their transformation is thought. By tracing thought to its origin, Reality is revealed.

The Reality that sustains and appears as relative reality, is stable and changeless, inexhaustible, life-affirming and infinitely blissful. Many of us have allowed our awareness to be reduced, circumscribed and conditioned by the framework of relative reality, and have forsaken our Wholeness. We can regain the limitless perspective of Reality and live from It consciously, while expressing and experiencing through the ever-changing world of relativity. Deep meditation and steady contemplation of Reality help restore us. The relative worlds are not to be overcome, but rather accorded with harmoniously, in the freedom of Being.

O

Belief systems and conceptual descriptions about Reality certainly cannot satisfy our inner hunger for conscious restoration with Reality (returning to Wholeness), but because such a hunger exists gives evidence that we are not actually apart from the Reality we seek. As Reality emerges, our hunger diminishes.

O

The perfection and completeness of Reality exist simultaneously throughout the time-space continuum. Wherever we are, Reality is. The more refined our powers of perception are, the more evident this is. We recognize that every place is a "sacred place" and that every being is Reality in expression.

While dreaming, we can experience the same degree of realness and range of emotions that we know while awake. Following a dream experience, we are sometimes surprised and even amused that the dream sequence seemed so realistic and that it affected us so strongly while we were immersed in it. Through the perspective of wakefulness, we recognize that our dreams are composites of creative thoughts, supported and fortified by our complete identification with them. We become fully invested in the personalities and interactions of those dream characters. Similarly, during waking consciousness, we tend to invest so completely in the portrayal of our conditioned mortal identity, in relation to the on-going world drama, that we forsake our innate capacity for limitless Awareness and conditionless Fulfillment, or Spiritual Wakefulness. When we are spiritually awake, we view our role of individuality and the continually changing scenes of the world stage as one imperishable Reality, enacting countless expressions of Itself. In this unbounded Awareness we can fully appreciate our participation in time and space, while also enjoying the cosmic perspective of changeless Awareness. In a sense, we can become Conscious dreamers.

O

Recognizing the Perpetual Impulse in life, gratitude awakens. Cooperating with this underlying, unifying Impulse brings the deepest fulfillment and the most worthy contribution. The active representation of this Benevolent Impulse is our deepest obligation and the way to liberation.

O

Gratitude naturally arises through the unobstructed recognition of what *is:* that all is perfectly ordered and unconditionally sanctioned. This is the realization of Abundance and the dawning of Contentment.

Meditation involvement requires a momentum of willed effort and willing effortlessness! Alertness and an enduring focus of attention are essential for success in meditation practice, yet our approach must be relaxed, with increasing self-surrender. The vital force that is customarily expended through outward pursuits is gathered internally and directed toward continual absorption in the chosen object of meditation. In time, the state of Meditative Awareness dawns spontaneously, as the common subject-object orientation is dispelled.

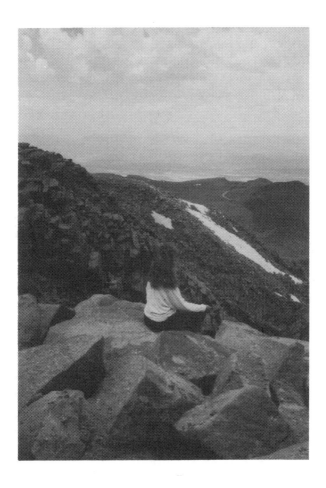

Though we may have glimpsed Reality, until we realize mind-body integrity, we still have work to do! Self-evolution occurs through degrees of self-integration, which is concerned with the resolution of psychophysiological conflicts, supported by spiritual awakening. Day by day we have the opportunity to more completely manifest our innate Wholeness in thought and action.

O

As we allow our sensitivity to increase, we are able to perceive ourselves and our world more completely. As we open ourselves in trust, being willing to see and feel more deeply, intuitive understanding is awakened. This is a state of quiet vulnerability that enables us to comprehend the underlying character of life: the Intelligent Impulse that supports all beings. By living sensitively, we cultivate internal strength and stability, comfortably established in the natural serenity and wisdom of our Being.

O

All vibrations of light and sound, and their multifaceted manifestations, issue from a Unified Field of silent stillness and are contained by It.

O

Enlightenment is not an all or nothing proposition—either you are or you're not! It is usually a process of progressive awakenings followed by periods of assimilation. Each of us experiences and expresses through various degrees of awareness and comprehension, which are transformed through time. We are operating from a different capacity of consciousness today than we did when we were younger. We have unfolded innate potentials to whatever level of actualization, through the years, and we can continue to do so. Likewise, enlightenment often occurs through degrees of unfoldment and can continue to mature through time.

O

In the spontaneous vision of Oneness, all vanity, pride and striving to become are dissolved. We see that all things are accomplished and every being is empowered.

The results of meditation are many, and they vary from person to person, according to temperament and need. Pure Meditation is the natural state or essential Being-nature of every person. To whatever degree this is realized during meditation practice, beneficial influences of health restoration, creative inspiration and enlightened insight are received.

O

In essence we are ever Whole, Complete and Content. We do not lack in any sense, for we are the perpetual Being that sustains all expressions of Itself. Operating through an individually conditioned mind-body, we take on the concept and sensation of being separate from the totality of life's multidimensional processes. We maintain an individual personality, exhibiting uniqueness, while harboring personal likes and dislikes, as we interact with others. The dilemma is that by identifying *exclusively* as an individualized expression, we forsake our Essential Fullness. Awakening, we recognize that we are the Eternal Being operating through individualized mind-body functioning, in order to express creatively and uniquely in time and space. We have entered into a grand drama in which we are but playing a part; a relative viewpoint of one perpetual Being. We are the oceanic Being, expressing as individualized wavelets. In this understanding we recognize the true Unity of all beings.

O

Through meditation practice, our awareness is released from the accustomed perspective of mind-body exclusiveness. We find that our awareness is independent of sensory perceptions, relative conditionings and thought activities, yet links and operates through these functions. We then recognize the possibility of living freely, within the mind-body continuum, while traversing the ordered cycles of time and space.

O

Life is a journey that is unique to each, yet common to all. We each share in a profound process that resolves more and more into Love. We have come into this life to live and express the Love that we are. Love is the supreme wisdom sanctioning life. Loving is the ultimate action performed through illumined minds.

Our current state of functional consciousness represents the cumulative process of personal growth (unfoldment). What we are today is the culmination of all we have experienced and thought. This is the relative perspective of self-development. What we are in Essence is above and not dependent on this process. What is seen as personal growth or self-development is actually the gradual uncovering of the innate purity of Consciousness that is our essential Self. The natural free functioning of Consciousness becomes more dominantly expressive as the mind is progressively cleared of conceptual restrictions.

O

The internal space between the eyebrows, known as the "Ajna Chakra," is a mystic center through which we may return to Full Awareness. This center is intimately linked with the pituitary gland and the function of refined intelligence and perception. It is here that the individualized self-consciousness unfolds into cosmic Self-consciousness. Within this center, subtle formations of light and the mixture of fine vibrational frequencies are perceived. By flowing attention continuously through this mystic gateway, the magnetic, attracting current of Spirit becomes predominant, and one-pointed focus is effortless. By merging with internal light, sound, and this redeeming current, we are lifted into Full Awareness.

O

Creative visualization can be used following meditation, as a complement to our efforts to live harmoniously and fully. After immersion in the peaceful contentment of meditation, we are likely to desire that which is enriching for everyone and that which conforms to the process of spiritual evolution. By envisioning what hasn't yet been, as though it now is, we help co-create relative circumstances.

O

To enter Transcendental Awareness, condense thought and awareness (feeling) by flowing attention upward through the internal spine, like a continuous fountain of warm liquid light. Be as one with this surging stream of radiant force and persist until there is no striving.

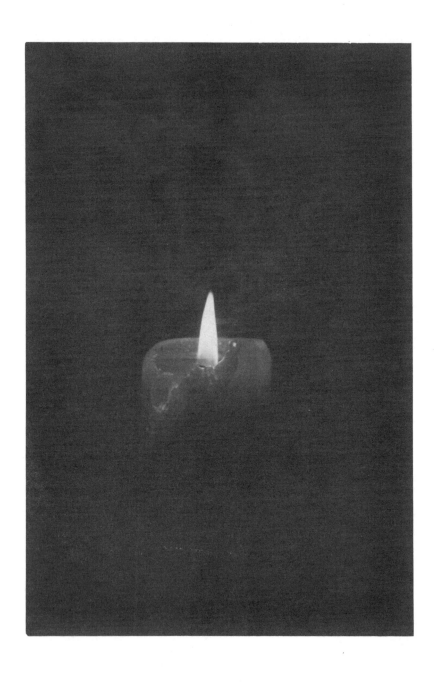

MEDITATIVE POETRY

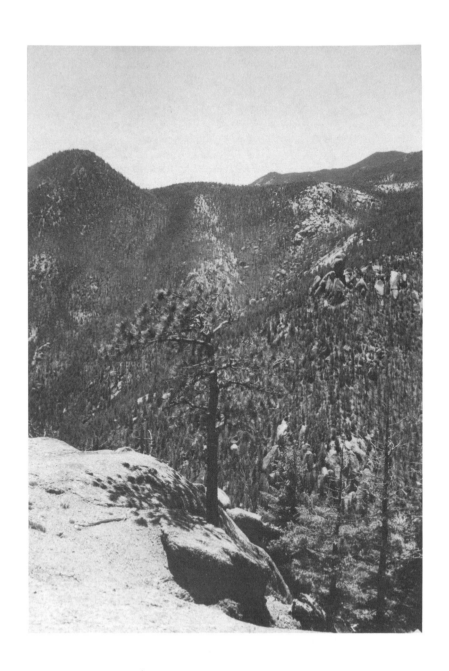

Observations of Nature

The serene eyes of the poet
Sensitively scan nature's responses
To the Benevolent Direction

Comforted by the intricate cycles
Continually at play,
Peace pervades

Nature flourishes, thrives and survives,
Willingly open to the unseen Nourisher

Each atom vibrates purposefully,
Contributing harmoniously . . .
Spherical dancing drama, on and on

Without differentiation
Perfection is reflected
In all Life's faces!

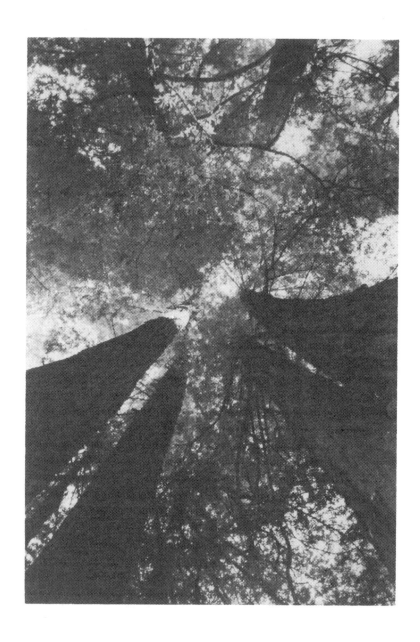

In nature
Returned to Being

Quiet and alone
With awe and wonder
As a child

The cricket symphony,
The deep darkening sky,
The friendly stars: ancient vaulted heavens
Familiar mystery: the puzzle of lifetimes

Comfortable,
Out of time . . .
Ah, the nowness of peace
In the Heart

Innocent . . .
Soft . . .
The tender life pulse

A perfect world
Everywhere at rest,
Effortlessly, the Creative Stream
Filling the universe,
OOOOOOOOMMMMMMMmmmmmmmmm . . .

—·—·—

                        Poetic fields of sparkling white,
                        Autumn's first!

                        Sun and clouds
                        Transform fluid crystal colonies
                        Effortlessly, nature's creative hands

                        Beneath accumulated blankets
                        Indistinct potentials patiently await
                        The freeing Light of spring.

                        —·—·—

Light flakes stack
And join

Sparkling white sculptures
Contour familiar gardens
At rest

In the tenderness
Of inner solitude,
Each new breath is birth!

—·—··—

                  Majestic landscapes,
                  Woven order and cooperation

                  A yielding peace,
                  An Essence merged in matter

                  In like vibration
                  Inner certainty resonates

                  Wholeness,
                  Our Reality.

—·—··—

Waterfall beauty,
Sequoia magnificence,
Effortless effort

Leaves sail,
Chimes freely sing

Life-death
Earth cycles.

—·—··—

Glistening new snow unifies
A forest community,
Pausing in renewal

Motionless pines
Meditate on icy slopes

A perpetual Force imperceptibly
Nurtures the many
In profound wisdom.

—·—·—

                Shrouded in winter,
                Patient pines humbly bow

                Stability in adversity,
                Enduring soft-strength!

—·—·—

Chaperones of hope and regret vanish,
In this stark wintery landscape,
Imprinting the mind with no-thought stillness

All stands frozen, between breaths
Aloft from appointment and disappointment,
Naked, with no striving

The impact of Now!
The expansive sobriety of seeing
No other.

—·—·—

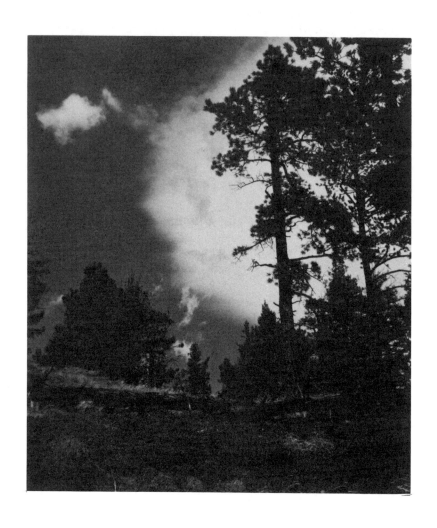

Perpetually sanctioned cycles,
Bearing seasons
Of life-giving dreams

Within time
All must seek

With and without time
ONE is.

Profound beauty
Of the moment . . .

Who can alertly receive it?

As quiet as an evening snowfall,
As serene as a redwood grove at dusk,
As still and expansive as star-blanketed skies of summer
And the purity of the dawning sun

The moment swells
To meet receptive ears

Love bursting
From the heart of each atom

Who can feel it?

— · — · —

        Surface impressions
        Of independent lives
        In perpetual motion,
        Escorted through unified cycles . . .

        The One and the Many
        Are ONE!

— · — · —

Internal Observations

Dividing into good and bad,
Spiritual—non-spiritual,
That which is now Perfect

Tarnished windows of perception,
Conditionings of life-cycles intact,
Of dreaming duality and becoming,
Deadens awareness-clarity-bliss

"Cleanliness is next to Godliness"
Because when we are really clean
Heaven is our perception.

———

Far from the competitive fervor,
Above maleness and femaleness,
A Peace pervades

The stillness of Being . . .
Beyond all wayward musing,
A perpetual field of Healing exists
For all to take refuge

The intellect can't know It
Nor can the body sense It,
Yet within us there is Radiance,
Boundless and ever pure,
That may be fully known, received and accorded with

Abandoning confines of concepts held,
There is Contentment without end . . .
A Completeness that surpasses every thing

This is the Abode from which we spring,
Ever at hand, when surrendered,
Its reality is our identity

Many seek in vain, dabbling with "the 10,000 things"
Yet how simple to be still and Know,
To lift the veil of lifetimes.

———

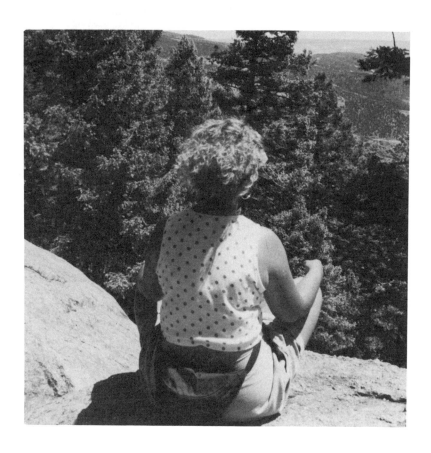

Unconscious hands clasp gently,
A grateful heart sings unspeakable joy . . .
Great Silence prevails

Creation vibrates gratitude,
Linking each atom . . .
The human symphony extends to Infinity

In breathless Unity,
We breathe again . . .
Cycles progress through timeless Light.

In the abode of The Most High,
There is no singing of hymns,
Chanting of mantras,
Recitation of prayers

Silent emanations of Peace radiate endlessly
In Communion.

──────

        Inside the time-space realms
        There is a sacred Place of no place

        Individual life-endowed complexities
        Revolve through roles, supported by universal precept

        Above and within this,
        A placeless Place endures, unrestricted

        The dissolving of heartaches, dreamscapes, inherited ways,
        Is effortless,
        Following arduous effort! (What dissolves?)

        Reflecting on Freedom
        Of and from . . .

        Doing within Being,
        Without doing

        Order woven through change . . .
        To dream becoming,
        Knowing it never was Actual

        Beholding One as all,
        Extending Peace to all.

──────

Stuff . . .
Inside—outside,
Only stuff!

Self,
Watching stuff parade . . .

Why add stuff to Self?

—·—·—

        Ageless wisdom-words surface,
        Healing our world

        The Teacher
        Forsaking the forsaking,
        Without gain or sacrifice

        Joyous fountain of service!

—·—·—

Indifferent to have and have not,
In a mind of quiet unity,
Distant from things,
With everything at hand

When Real
We live in no-birth, all-birth Love

None are deluded,
None are striving . . .
All are Love

—·—·—

How far do we stray,
Like windblown leaves of autumn?

Pain-driven passions
Within the dream continuum
Of thought-formed worlds

Being danced by the Grand Host
Of conceptual strivings

Shadowed memories of the Spirit-Heart,
Prospering us, while awaiting our return.

—·—·—

                        Meditation works its magic . . .
                        With absorption,
                        The Source pervades
                        Conceptual mansions of mind stuff

                        Bathed in Peace,
                        Permeated with Comfort,
                        Encircled by Love . . .
                        Inside-out,
                        I AM.

—·—·—

Awakening to enter
The solitude of early morning meditation

Awareness flows
Through increasingly subtle recesses
As peacefulness engulfs worldliness
With soothing welcome

Secure and stable
Amidst the trauma of dreams.

—·—·—

Forgetting all we have built and become
And strived for . . .

We can recall the Purity
The Reality

The freedom of Being
As we are.

— - — - —

                Contemplating . . .
                In Stillness,
                Motion and change
                Reveal their nature

                Stillness contains
                Flux and transformation,
                Where universes, fine to gross,
                Issue and fade

                Can you be Still
                And know your Original Name?

— - — - —

No words,
Emptying into no thought
Samadhi stillness

Peace rebirth
Extinguishes desire worlds
In cosmic stability

The profound simplicity
In Wakefulness.

— - — - —

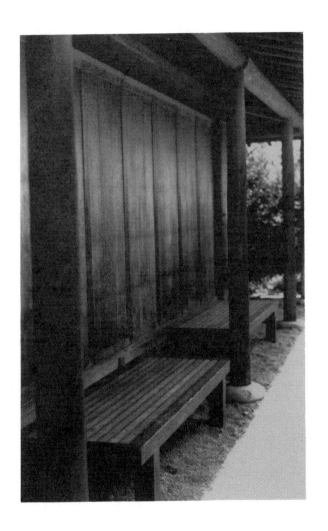

AUTHOR'S NOTE

The meditation methods offered here are simple, direct and effective, though they do not replace the beneficial guidance of personal instruction. Engage in these practices calmly, conforming exactly to the instructions without deviation or embellishment and the stated results will occur. The key to success is to practice regularly and correctly with patience.

You may contact the author directly to receive clarification on matters related to your meditation practice and for information about his workshop programs, as well as any concerns regarding the material presented in this book.

>Steve Ridley
>1921 Jasmine St.
>Denver, CO 80220

APPENDIX

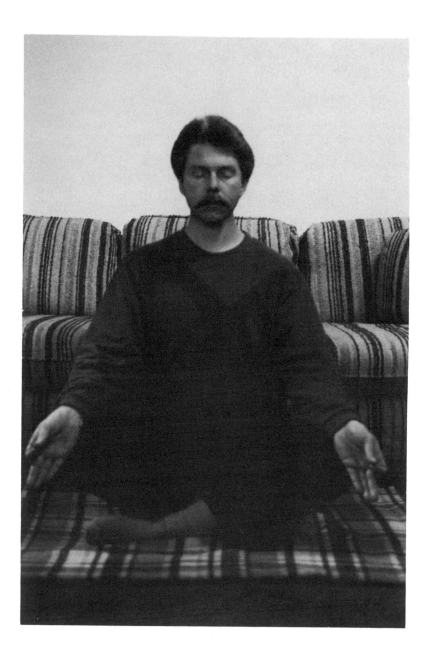

General Meditation Instruction

The ultimate objectives of meditation practice are to awaken to the direct cognition of our Original Consciousness and to integrate this Actual Identity wholly, through the mind-body, in order to actualize our fullest potentials for creative and responsible living. When Original Consciousness is our dominant perspective, we are joyously content and usefully active. Through sincere and consistent practice of meditation, these ultimate objectives will be realized.

The following method of meditation is tried and proven. It will result in success if applied properly and persistently, through time. The use of this technique helps arrange the psychophysiological environment so that it is conducive to Pure Meditation.

Practice once or twice each day for 15 to 30 minutes, in a clean, quiet space with good ventilation. Sit upright with spine and head in alignment, either in a chair or on the floor, being relaxed and alertly focused on the process.

Preparation:

1) Even Breathing: Breathe in slowly at one speed, evenly, filling the lungs completely, without strain. Retain the breath for a like duration, remaining relaxed. Exhale slowly, at one speed, and gently contract the abdominal muscles at the conclusion. Repeat this process continually for 10 to 20 rounds.

2) Tensing-Relaxing: Inhale quickly, filling the lungs. Retain the breath while lightly tensing every muscle, simultaneously, for three seconds. Exhale forcefully through the mouth, relaxing every muscle at once. Repeat this process three times and rest, being still and completely at ease.

Concentration Technique:

3) Internal Focus: Flow your attention continually through the internal space between the eyebrows, remaining calmly centered. Feel that this space is a delicate membrane through which you can sense the passage of breath, as it naturally occurs. Resting stably at this interior center, feel the in-breath and out-breath as they spontaneously issue, without regulation of the process. Simply witness the passage of breath, sensitively, as though it is taking place through the internal forehead center. When there are natural pauses between breaths, continue to rest alertly within this center, until the next breath occurs.

In addition to this method of focus, introduce the mental recitation of "OM" as each breath flows in and "PEACE" as each breath flows out, as though the sound is emanating from the center of focus. Continue with this technique until the conclusion of your practice period or until the technique is transcended and Pure Meditation is realized, to whatever degree.

Following Meditation:

4) Integration: After each meditation practice period, continue to sit quietly and affirm: "I am spiritually awake, mentally alert and physically strong." Open the eyes and breathe deeply several times, including the immediate environment in your awareness. Be thankful and happy.

Regardless of mental impressions and emotional surges that may surface during practice, be steadfast and alert in your focus of attention. When you find that your concentration is faltering, take a deep breath, exhale forcefully through the mouth and begin anew. Above all, be patient with yourself and persist. This method will eventually reveal the innate Original Consciousness that is ever pure and complete.

Tan T'ien Meditation

The tan t'ien is the vital center in the lower portion of the abdomen where chi is accumulated and stored through T'ai Chi practice and mental focus. This center is directly related to the functions of procreation, regeneration and, in general, the promotion of vitality. By focusing attention on the tan t'ien, chi is gathered and developed there, and all related physiological processes benefit. Through continual mental absorption at this center, profound Meditation can be experienced. The following is a simple meditation practice that can be utilized as a prelude to sleep for rejuvenation and mystical insight.

Procedure:

1) Lie down on your back with legs straight and heels touching. Rest the palms lightly on the lower abdomen, with thumbtips on either side of the navel and index fingertips touching just above the pubic bone, the rest of the fingers gathered together. This position creates an open triangular space, framing the tan t'ien, which is said to reside "three finger widths below the navel and two finger widths inside."

2) Relax completely and maintain your hand position. Direct your attention to the tan t'ien by subtly tuning into the sensation there, using feeling to place your awareness within the center. Mentally reside within the tan t'ien with an attitude of calm alertness.

3) Focus awareness on the spontaneous breathing process by noticing each inhalation and exhalation as it occurs. Assume and feel that each inhalation is being drawn in through the space below the navel, and that each exhalation is passing out through that space. Continue to observe and feel each breath in this way, without regulating breathing patterns. Persist in this manner until you enter sleep.

Along with the cultivation of chi at the tan t'ien through concentrated focus of attention, authentic revelations can dawn. You may experience a vast continuum of creative energy, have subtle realizations about the nature of this evolutionary force, or enjoy a more dynamic expression of it as it circulates in greater volume to quicken healing and spiritual awakening.

To derive the fullest benefits of this specialized practice, repeat it each night without fail, prior to sleep, for at least one month, regardless of results.

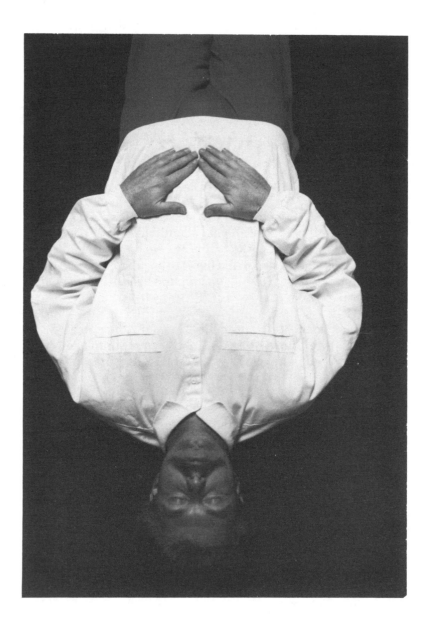

Meditation to Awaken the Heart Center

Meditation on the Heart Center or "Anahata Chakra" will banish fear, summon courage and awaken expansive awareness. This center is directly linked to the functioning of the thymus gland and regulation of the immune system, and it is where selflessness, compassion and unconditional love are developed.

To activate the Heart Center, sit or stand with hands placed in a prayerful position ("Salutation Mudra") at the sternum. Breathe slowly, evenly and completely for several minutes while concentrating deeply within this center, being relaxed and steady in your posture. Once your concentration is established, begin to produce the continuous sound of 'AH' while slowly exhaling, by placing the vibration in the chest cavity. Repeat this sound over and over again, allowing its vibration to expand and project effortlessly from the Heart Center, until it seems you are no longer initiating the sound. Then relax and be still with your awareness absorbed within the Heart Center, beyond technique and striving. Rest in silence.

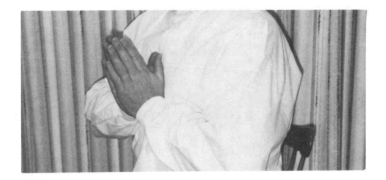

For a complete catalog of related materials, please contact:

Good Karma Publishing, Inc.
P.O. Box 511
Fort Yates, ND 58538
701/854-7459